Thyroid Diseases, Conditions, Autoimmunity and Cancers

Disorders Affecting
the Metabolic Butterfly

TABLE OF CONTENTS:

INTRODUCTION:

There are many diseases that affect thyroid function, including those that cause hypothyroidism, hyperthyroidism, thyroid swelling (goiter), tumors in the gland (nodules), thyroid eye disease and thyroid cancer. When this small, butterfly-shaped gland becomes imbalanced in its function, bodily metabolism is affected. In this book I will present information on these conditions of thyroid dysfunction and the diseases that cause them including thyroid autoimmunity.

The subjects addressed in the chapters that follow, include signs and symptoms of thyroid disorders, their diagnosis and treatments. Types of goiters, nodules and cancers of the thyroid gland are also discussed in addition to pharmaceutical and surgical procedures for treating them and post-op treatments.

I, Jim Lowrance was Editor for Thyroid Health at a major content website and moderator for the associated patient support forum, during years 2008 and 2009. I was awarded Editor's Choice Awards for general health articles written for Suite101.com, during years 2010 and 2011.

Thyroid Diseases, Conditions, Autoimmunity and Cancers

It is my hope that this book proves to be a good general educational resource for its readers on diseases and conditions affecting the thyroid gland.

CHAPTER ONE

Thyroid Autoimmunity

The majority of patients with both hypothyroidism (underactive thyroid) and hyperthyroidism (overactive thyroid) are experiencing autoimmune diseases that cause these conditions. When autoimmune thyroid disease results in hypothyroidism, the term for the disease is "Hashimoto's thyroiditis." When the autoimmune disease of the thyroid causes hyperthyroidism, it is called "Grave's Disease." In this chapter, I will be presenting information in regard to Hashimoto's thyroiditis, with more on Graves' disease in a later chapter.

The immune system normally sends out antibodies, which are killer cells, to eradicate foreign invaders from the body that can make us sick. These invaders include viruses, bacteria and allergens. The purpose of antibodies is to seek these out and destroy them, so as to prevent our bodies from becoming ill. The problem with "thyroid antibodies" is that, like other antibodies that cause autoimmune diseases, they are directed against the thyroid gland as if it is one of these invaders.

It is a case of mistaken identity that over time causes damage to the thyroid gland and ongoing cell death. Eventually, the antibodies will disable the thyroid gland completely.

The Search for Causes and Cures of Autoimmune Disease Continues

Medical research is ongoing; to better understand conditions of autoimmunity (autoimmune diseases) so that hopefully, treatment for the immune root-cause can reverse them. Several theories have evolved through studies by medical groups including the opinion that autoimmune diseases might possibly be triggered by viral infections that are experienced during childhood, that cause autoimmune responses in later life.

I personally have expressed the opinion in previous articles I have written, in regard to the possibility that when permanently carried viruses cannot be fully eradicated by the immune system, it eventually turns on the body. Some organs of the body such as the thyroid gland, the kidneys, the liver or even the muscles in-general, that hold concentrated amounts of viruses, may be targeted by the immune system.

They are seen as enemies in the body, due to an inability by the immune system to rid the body of these foreign cells they contain, that typically cause illness in healthy tissues.

It is also a fact that people with dysfunctional immune systems or those that are compromised by disease processes in the body can begin to loose the ability to adequately suppress the replication of viruses in the body. In Chronic Fatigue Syndrome patients for example, it has been found that viruses such as EBV (Epstein - Barr virus), Human Herpes Virus 6 (HHV-6) and more recently the Murine Leukemia Virus (MLV - XMRV) are found in high titers (blood lab measurements) in their blood. This indicates that the immune system is failing to hold the virus at bay as it should and high levels begin to infiltrate the deeper tissues of the body.

Epstein-Barr Virus in Autoimmune Diseases

Approximately 80% of the general population is infected with EBV. Even when immunity against EBV initially develops in a person's body, the dormant virus can later go on to cause the onset of chronic, autoimmune or inflammatory diseases in susceptible individuals.

The virus is also linked to causing certain types of cancer. The initial illness of Mononucleosis (mono) that can result from EBV infection is usually not serious or life-threatening but the viral symptoms of fatigue, body aches and swollen lymph nodes in the neck will require bed rest, increased fluid intake and over-the-counter anti-inflammatory drugs to moderate fever. This illness, also referred to as "the kissing disease" usually resolves within six weeks of contracting it. Many people, who contract the virus and carry it in their bodies lifelong, do not experience the symptoms of mono. Even with this being the case, this particular virus is far more hazardous to public health than was previously believed for roughly the past 30 years.

Medical authorities in the past believed that everyone infected with EBV becomes immune to it, with no re-occurrence from it of any kind or complications in it affecting the immune system. There was also previously very little research in regard to it causing other diseases but for the past several years, this belief has drastically changed. They now agree that the virus "reactivates" and "replicates" in some people and goes-on to cause or at least contribute-to the development of many other diseases.

Thyroid Diseases, Conditions, Autoimmunity and Cancers

The EBV virus is "significantly" more common in autoimmune thyroiditis patients and in Sjogren's Syndrome patients, than in healthy patients, according to research articles published on the National Institutes of Health/National Library of Medicine website (PubMed). You can find this research in articles titled: *"Epstein-Barr virus serology in patients with autoimmune thyroiditis"* and *"Association of Epstein-Barr virus (EBV) with Sjögren's syndrome: differential EBV expression between epithelial cells and lymphocytes in salivary glands"*.

Another research article of interest in this area is titled: *"DIAGNOSTICS AND THERAPY OF EPSTEIN-BARR VIRUS IN AUTOIMMUNE DISORDERS"*. This research, found on the "World Intellectual Property Organization" website, states that "The Oklahoma Medical Research Foundation", is trying to develop a vaccine for EBV following a filed patent on their proposed intellectual formula for one. The firm's research states the fact that a vaccine is needed due to the EBV reactivating in some immune-deficient people, causing autoimmune diseases.

In an article found on the "Medical News Today", online magazine, titled: *"Epstein-Barr Virus Might Kick-start Multiple Sclerosis"* (May 7, 2006), they also refer to research on the association between Multiple Sclerosis and EBV.

In an article on the "Lymphoma Information Network" website, they state that EBV is associated with Hodgkins Disease (lymphoma cancer) and is found present in the blood samples of 40% to 60% of patients with Hodgkins.

EBV is also common in people with Lupus Erythematosus (SLE). It remains dormant or latent in these particular people but can reactivate and becomes a possible trigger for development of Lupus, according to the "arthritis Foundation", in their article titled: *"Epstein-Barr virus and lupus"*.

In an article on the "BioMed Central" website titled: *"Epstein-Barr virus load in rheumatoid arthritis patients and normal controls: accurate quantification using real time PCR"*, it states that medical research has identified EBV as a cause of Rheumatoid Arthritis, which they have suspected for over 20 years.

Thyroid Diseases, Conditions, Autoimmunity and Cancers

According to the "Clinical Cancer Research" website, EBV has been implemented as a cause of Burkitt's lymphoma, Hodgkin's disease (previously mentioned), non-Hodgkin's lymphoma, nasopharyngeal carcinoma, and lymphomas, as well as leiomyosarcomas, some of these, being forms of cancer.

EBV can be a trigger for autoimmune hepatitis, as is discussed in the article found on the "CAT.INIST" website (European scientific research catalog), titled: *"Epstein-Barr virus as a trigger for autoimmune hepatitis in susceptible individuals"*.

Evidence of Epstein-Barr virus affecting mucosal inflammatory cells of ulcerative colitis, is found on the "PubMed" website in a research article titled *"Evidence of Epstein-Barr virus infection in ulcerative colitis."*

EBV antibodies are associated with neurological diseases as well, including; Bell's palsy, encephalitis and acute cerebellar ataxia, according to a page on the PubMed website titled: *"Epstein-Barr virus antibodies in neurological diseases"*.

They also discuss this in their article titled: *"Antibodies to Epstein-Barr virus in neurological diseases"*, which states that the infected person may never have had mononucleosis but is still carrying the EB Virus.

Many of these articles, including the last one I refer to above, clearly state that EBV does not have to manifest as mono at any point in a person's life, to cause these problems and that the virus can "reactivate" and "replicate" in some carriers. This is not hype, this EBV research is vast and ultra-reputable. This virus may be one of the most prominent factors in causing autoimmune diseases that exists.

It is incredible that they are only lately trying to develop a vaccine for EBV. The number of diseases, including autoimmune ones that it is believed EBV can cause, including those that are thyroid-related, such as Hashimoto's thyroiditis is alarming.

The Diagnosis of Hashimoto's thyroiditis

"Hashimoto's thyroiditis" is also referred to as "chronic lymphocytic thyroiditis" and is the most common cause of hypothyroidism, in the U.S. and other industrialized countries. Patients suspected of having this autoimmune form of thyroid disease, need to be tested for "thyroid antibodies", in addition to being tested for low levels of thyroid hormone. The antibody tests can reveal autoimmune thyroid disease going on, in patients with normal-range thyroid hormone levels.

The tests that help detect Hashimoto's thyroiditis, are the "anti-TPO" (anti-thyroidperoxidase), "anti-TG" (anti-thyroglobulin) and sometimes also the "TSI" antibodies (thyroid stimulating immunoglogulin). People with developing autoimmune hypothyroidism (Hashimoto's thyroiditis), can have elevated antibody levels that cause symptoms, even with thyroid hormones within normal-range.

Medical research articles by reputable research groups, state that the disease process itself, caused by thyroid antibodies can be a factor in causing symptoms in Hashimoto's patients.

These research articles conclude that elevated levels of these antibodies can cause fibromyalgia type symptoms in persons with only sub-clinical hypothyroidism. Other medical-source articles state that the autoimmune thyroid disease can have a degree of systemic (system wide) effect as well, so that the over activity of the immune system affects not only the thyroid gland area but other parts of the body as well.

Patients with Hashimoto's thyroiditis can also go through phases of hyperthyroidism, before the onset of progressive hypothyroidism sets in and the term for this related condition is "Hashitoxicosis". These patients are the ones mentioned previously, who might need to be blood tested for "TSI antibodies" because the hyperthyroid phases they go through, are due to having these antibodies, that normally cause Grave's Disease (autoimmune hyperthyroidism), in addition to having the ones that typically cause Hashimoto's thyroiditis.

You could almost say that these type patients are suffering from Grave's and Hashimoto's, simultaneously.

Even without having the TSI antibodies present, Hashimoto's patients can still experience spells of thyroiditis, which can cause mild hyperthyroid type symptoms that are not as severe as those caused by Hashitoxicosis but that are still concerning.

Treatment for Hashimoto's thyroiditis

There is actually no treatment for the thyroiditis caused by auto-antibodies from the immune system. However, once the thyroid gland begins to under-function (hypothyroidism), due to damage from being attacked by these thyroid antibodies, it cannot usually be reversed and the patient will have to begin thyroid hormone replacement medication that will most likely be a lifelong treatment. (More in regard to hypothyroid therapy, via replacement hormone will be addressed in the next chapter.)

There are temporary types of thyroiditis, that can present similar to Hashimoto's but these type resolve within a few weeks or a couple months period of time and the patient's blood results will not show an elevation of the thyroid antibodies that cause permanent, autoimmune thyroiditis.

Short term thyroiditis can also first manifest with a phase of hyperthyroidism as Hashimoto's can but afterward, hypothyroid symptoms do not occur as they do with permanent thyroiditis, which results in progressive hypothyroidism that must eventually be treated when it reaches an overt state (detectable via blood tests and symptom-manifestations).

In very rare cases, Hashimoto's will reverse and the antibodies will diminish, before permanent damage to the thyroid has occurred but for the vast majority of Hashimoto's patients, the autoimmune process continues to damage the thyroid, eventually resulting in the need for hormone replacement therapy. Hashimoto's is not a temporary form of Thyroiditis but a chronic, permanent form.

As hypothyroidism occurs in patients with Hashimoto's, they begin to experience the symptoms of an under active thyroid.

These may include:

• *Tiredness, fatigue, lack of energy and stamina*

• *Depressed mood, at times alternating with anxiety*

- - -

- *Dry skin that flakes and dry brittle hair that tends to fall out*
- *Constipation from slowed digestion*
- *Slowed heart rate, hypotension and at times hypertension*
- *Moderate weight gain from slowed metabolism*
- *Goiter or nodules of the thyroid*
- *Joint & muscle aches and stiffness*

Joint & Muscle Pain

Patients with Hashimoto's complain of the symptoms listed above but one of the more concerning symptoms, is mild to moderate "joint and muscle pain". What aspect of this disease, results in the concerning symptoms that affect the patient's joints and muscles? There are many contributing factors however, I believe two of the main causes, are inflammation and decreased blood circulation, from slowed metabolism. The inflammatory aspect is from the autoimmune process of antibodies attacking the thyroid gland, resulting in high levels of inflammation.

The inflammation first affects the area of the thyroid gland itself but it is my belief, that over time, continuing inflammation is going to eventually have a degree of systemic affect (not staying localized in the thyroid gland) and travel to other parts of the body.

I also believe it is no coincidence that some autoimmune disease thyroid patients often complain of their joint pain, first manifesting more severely, in their shoulders and cervical (upper) spine area. These are the joints that are closest to the thyroid. Over time, these joint pains can spread to other areas of the body, sometimes all the way down to the feet and all the way out to the fingertips. This can lead patients and doctors to suspect fibromyalgia as the cause, until diagnostic tests reveal thyroid disease.

Hypothyroid Neuropathies

Patients may also experience nervous system involvement in their rheumatic symptoms. Following are five research quotes regarding neuro-muscular symptoms in hypothyroid patients:

- - -

1. *Pain and small-fiber neuropathy in patients with hypothyroidism* (U.S. National Library of Medicine – PubMed) --- "Conclusions: Some patients treated for hypothyroidism have symptoms and findings compatible with small-fiber neuropathy or "hyper phenomena" indicating central sensitization. ...of Eighteen patients...Eight were classified as having large fiber neuropathy..."

2. *Hypothyroidism and polyneuropathy.* (U.S. National Library of Medicine – PubMed) --- "Using standard electrophysiological criteria, a definite diagnosis of polyneuropathy was made in 28 cases (72%). The commonest sites of abnormal nerve conduction were the sensory nerves, especially the sural nerve."

3. *Hypothyroid neuropathy and myopathy: clinical and electrodiagnostic longitudinal findings.* (U.S. National Library of Medicine – PubMed) --- "This case shows that thyroid hormone replacement eliminates the neuropathic manifestations of severe hypothyroidism. In contrast, the myopathic features, such as weakness and muscle wasting, may persist despite maintenance of the euthyroid state."

4. *Neuromuscular status of thyroid diseases: a prospective clinical and electrodiagnostic study.* (U.S. National Library of Medicine – PubMed) --- Among the thyroid patients, 17 (42.5%) patients were diagnosed with mononeuropathy and polyneuropathy. Entrapment neuropathy was observed in 30% and diffuse neuropathy in 10% of the patients. Myopathy findings were observed in 2 patients.

5. *Aspects of peripheral nerve involvement in patients with treated hypothyroidism.* (U.S. National Library of Medicine – PubMed) --- "RESULTS: Sixty-three per cent of the patients with 'pure' hypothyroidism had abnormalities on NCS, 25% had reduced IENF density and 31% had abnormalities on QST. Four patients (25%) met criteria for small fibre polyneuropathy, the other (75%) were classified as having mixed fiber polyneuropathy.

When neuropathy and/or myopathy symptoms continue in a patient that has been well-treated for thyroid hormone imbalance, other causes should be investigated by the treating doctor.

Different types of nutritional deficiencies can present with neuro-muscular symptoms, including vitamin, mineral, protein and electrolyte deficiencies. When these types of problems are found, treatments for them, via replacement therapies, can resolve them and can better-potentiate (aid in the effectiveness) thyroid hormone replacement therapy. Vitamins and minerals that are often found deficient in thyroid patients include vitamins B12 and D and the essential minerals – magnesium and selenium. Iron deficiency anemia can also develop if iron levels become low due to hypothyroidism.

CHAPTER TWO

Thyroid Hormone Replacement Therapy

The treatment for hypothyroidism caused by Hashimoto's thyroiditis is simply to "replace" the low thyroid hormone. This is done by giving the patient "thyroid hormone replacement medication". The Doctor will prescribe a starting dose for the patient and do follow-up blood re-testing to adjust the dose to the correct level over time, which is called "titrating, the dose".

The AACE (Thyroid Specialists) and other medical authorities recommend that hypothyroid patient's TSH levels while on thyroid hormone replacement medication, should be suppressed down to between "1.0 and 2.0". The average normal values range at blood testing labs is approximately between "0.5 and 5.0" but this may vary slightly,between labs. The TSH level rises, when thyroid hormone decreases with hypothyroidism and it falls below normal when the thyroid hormone level increases or with "hyperthyroidism".

If a patient's TSH is not kept below 2.0, they risk continued hypothyroid symptoms and if it is brought significantly below 1.0, patients are at risk for developing hyperthyroid symptoms. The main goal of thyroid hormone replacement therapy is to relieve the symptoms of hypothyroidism by normalizing the thyroid hormones (euthroid state) and if possible, optimizing them.

My Personal Experience with Hypothyroid Therapy

"Levothyroxine" is the name for synthetic T4 hormone replacement medication, which comes in the different brands such as "Synthroid, Levoxyl, Levothroid" etc... They are basically the same thing but some of these are considered generics and many doctors prefer to stick to the major brands, due to generics sometimes being less potent at same dose-levels. As a hypothyroid patient, I personally was started on Synthroid but didn't experience the expected relief of symptoms, so my Doctor placed me on a combination T3/T4 prescription hormone brand called "Armour Thyroid", which is a natural version, made from animal thyroid glands – porcine/pigs.

Natural brands of thyroid hormone are used for the same thing that the synthetic types are which is to restore normal hormone levels for hypothyroid patients.

The Doctor, who first treated me for hypothyroidism, switched me from the synthetic T4 only brand I had been taking for about a year, thinking I might have a problem with "T4 to T3 conversion" (a process that occurs naturally in the body but fails to do so in some patients). He switched me, believing I might be a person with the inability to convert T4 only hormone into the other needed T3 (more active) hormone, due to my experiencing unrelieved symptoms, while being on the Synthroid brand hormone.

Most people don't experience a problem with this and looking back I have a suspicion that mine was more of an "insufficient dosing" problem rather than an "impaired conversion" one because my blood TSH level (test used to monitor the therapy) was not suppressed adequately by my replacement therapy dose. Reputable medical sources state that TSH is supposed to be brought down (suppressed) to between 1.0 and 2.0 for proper treatment to occur.

Mine was only suppressed down to between 3.0 and 5.0 for at least that first year I was treated and the lower TSH level resulted in better symptom-relief in my case.

Natural Thyroid Supplements?

There are natural ways to compliment or what you might call "supplementing" your hypothyroid therapy but none of these are a substitute for thyroid hormone replacement therapy. For example, a healthy diet, exercise and healthy supplements (i.e. vitamins and safe well-researched health supplements containing no-iodine) can help, being careful to take those that contain calcium or iron, at least six hours apart from thyroid hormone dose (to prevent malabsorption they may cause). There are medical studies published by the U.S. NIH (PubMed) stating that "selenium" supplementation can reduce antibody levels and activity (i.e. inflammation and selling) in cases of autoimmune hypothyroidism. I do however believe-in running any supplements past a person's treating doctor, to help determine their safety.

As far as something that can substitute thyroid hormone replacement, there simply is <u>nothing that can do this</u> because the body absolutely requires it. It is also important that patients are assured by their doctors that treatment has been best-possible optimized. Doctors can do this by going over follow-up blood retests showing where their patient's thyroid hormone levels are as a result of their hormone therapy.

(More about Graves' disease and its treatment will be given in CHAPTER FOUR.)

CHAPTER THREE

Hashimoto's Encephalopathy Rare but Serious

There is a neuro-endocrine disorder that causes very serious and potentially life threatening symptoms, called Hashimoto's Encephalopathy (HE). The disorder can occur in patients with Hashimoto's thyroiditis, who experience a very high elevation of "thyroid antibody" levels. These antibodies, that attack the thyroid gland after recognition of it by the immune system, as a foreign invader, can become highly elevated in these rare cases of HE. At these high elevations they will begin to affect brain and nerve function in the body or the "neurological system" by causing inflammation in them. Severe symptoms will result because this system is the body's information and communication center and a disruption from a disease process can cause an array of nerve and brain related symptoms.

Inflammation caused by the antibodies (also called auto-antibodies) spreads to the brain and begins to affect the tissue containing the nerves that control bodily functions and impulses throughout the body.

The resulting effect, are severe neurological symptoms, meaning abnormal responses and manifestations of nervous system dysfunction.

These symptoms can include:

• *psychotic episodes - hallucinations and delusions*

• *dementia - mental deterioration*

• *neuropathies - abnormal nerve sensations*

• *coma or death if left untreated*

The antibodies responsible for causing thyroid destruction and inflammation in the thyroid gland but that can also cause HE when highly elevated, are the TPO and TG antibodies as previously described. This autoimmune disease called Hashimoto's thyroiditis that can result in the less common Hashimoto's Encephalopathy, is more often a result of elevated anti-TPO levels although it can result from elevations of both it and the anti-TG antibodies.

Thyroid hormone levels are not usually a factor in this potentially serious neuro-endocrine disorder of thyroid autoimmunity.

Some patients in fact have been documented in medical research, to have experienced HE with their thyroid hormone levels in normal range and before they were in need of thyroid hormone replacement therapy.

This disorder is a rare but a strong example of the fact that thyroid antibodies have the ability to produce bodily symptoms regardless of thyroid hormone levels.

Treatment for HE, is to reduce the inflammation caused by the thyroid antibodies by administering a steroid anti-inflammatory drug to patients who are diagnosed. These drugs, also called corticosteroids or hydrocortisone, mimic the anti-inflammatory properties of our body's own natural anti-inflammatory called "cortisol".

A major brand prescribed for inflammatory conditions is "Prednisone", a powerful steroid that usually achieves an anti-inflammatory effect quickly with only a relatively short term regimen of a few weeks being necessary to correct cases of HE.

If a patient with Hashimoto's thyroiditis or their loved ones, notice the onset of sudden and severe neurological symptoms, they should report to their Doctor immediately, to rule out HE as the cause. A delay in treatment for a patient experiencing this very rare disorder could result in irreversible damage to the brain and/or nervous system.

CHAPTER FOUR

Grave's Disease and Hyperthyroid Treatments

Some statistics estimate that over three million Americans suffer from Graves' disease and possibly as many as five million. This thyroid disorder which causes hyperthyroidism (over-active thyroid gland) is the result of an autoimmune response that sends out antibodies that attach to receptors in the thyroid gland.

Hyperthyroidism is a term simply meaning an overactive thyroid gland. The metabolism of a person with hyperthyroidism is sped up from too much thyroid hormone in their system, so that everything in the body is running at overdrive. When this happens, the person will experience hyperthyroid symptoms.

The symptoms of hyperthyroidism may include:

- *Rapid heart rate*
- *Hyperventilation*
- *Hypertension*
- *Excessive sweating*
- *Inability to sleep*

- - -

- *Nervousness and anxiety*
- *Diarrhea*
- *Excessive energy followed by fatigue*
- *Hair loss*
- *Weight loss*
- *Swelling of the thyroid gland (goiter)*

Patients who develop Graves' disease can have several antibodies directed against their thyroid glands. The antibodies cause destruction of the gland, plus swelling and goiter from resulting inflammation. The type of antibody that contributes to the hyper-functioning of the gland, however, is the "TSI" antibody (Thyroid Stimulating Immunoglobulin).

These specific antibodies are the ones that help to better diagnose a hyperthyroid patient as having Graves' disease. TSI antibodies are detected in a patient using blood lab testing. The vast majority of people with hyperthyroidism (95%) have Grave's Disease as the cause. This is an autoimmune disease caused by the antibodies described , created by the immune system that attach to the thyroid gland.

They stimulate it to produce excessive amounts of hormone by mimicking the stimulating properties of TSH (Thyroid Stimulating Hormone).

Most people with Grave's Disease have "toxic diffuse goiters", meaning they have an enlarged thyroid that is also over-producing hormones. These type goiters are also commonly painful in newly diagnosed Grave's patients. This disease can also have complications and co-morbid conditions occurring with it, including one called "Thyroid Eye Disease" (TED) an inflammatory condition that can cause swelling and bulging of the eyes and possible loss of vision, if not treated as early as possible. If hyperthyroidism caused by Grave's Disease goes untreated, serious health problems can develop including the following three major complications.

• *heart disease*

• *organ damage from hypertension*

• *chronic osteoporosis*

Treatment for Grave's Disease

Anti-thyroid medications are used to slow production of thyroid hormones. The thyroid gland produces mainly the "T-4 and T-3" hormones, but people with GD will have increased production of these as a result of the auto-antibodies that causes the disease. Patients will be given a trial of an anti-thyroid medication, which is designed to slow down the overactive thyroid so that thyroid hormones fall within normal values. Two of the more common brands of anti-thyroid medications are Methimazole (Tapazole) and Propylthiouracil (PTU).

Beta-blocker medications may also be used to control some of the symptoms of hyperthyroidism caused by GD. Beta-blockers, commonly prescribed for high blood pressure, are drugs that block the effects of adrenaline, the hormone sent out by the adrenal gland that helps stimulate heart rate and blood pressure regulation.

Patients with GD may have increased heart rate (tachycardia) and increased blood pressure (hypertension).

Administration of a beta-blocker as part of their treatment regimen may sometimes be used to control these abnormally high functioning bodily responses. Some GD patients may only be treated with a beta-blocker or only with an anti-thyroid medication, while some may be treated with both medications simultaneously.

Patients who have GD that cannot be controlled well using oral medications may need their thyroid gland surgically removed or destroyed through radioactive iodine treatment. When a GD sufferer has severe symptoms that are difficult to resolve, their doctor may refer them to a surgeon for partial or total removal of their thyroid gland. The names for these surgeries are "Total Thyroidectomy" (entire gland removal) and "Subtotal Thyroidectomy" (partial gland removal). Once this surgery has been performed, there is less or none of the thyroid gland in the patient's body to continue over-producing thyroid hormones.

The same is true of radioactive iodine treatment (also called "ablation" or "RAI") that is used to destroy the thyroid gland, rather than removing it surgically.

Patients afterward have no thyroid gland in their bodies and so they become hypothyroid (low thyroid hormone) following removal or ablation. With both types of thyroid removal treatments, the patient will have to be replaced lifelong with the missing hormone, through "Thyroid Hormone Replacement Therapy" medication.

Can Hyperthyroidism be resolved with Drug Treatment Only?

The answer/reply that follows below, was to a question posted to me by a hyperthyroid patient who was treated with an anti-thyroid drug only (NeoMercazole) and afterward they were placed on thyroid hormone replacement (Eltroxin) for hypothyroidism. It is actually rare for hyperthyroid cases to not require destruction or removal of the thyroid gland and is one of several points I made in my comments to them that follow. ---

My Reply:

"The drug NeoMercazole that you referred to in your question is an antithyroid medication that slows thyroid hormone production in an overactive gland.

With your hyperthyroidism resolving with this medication and not also requiring thyroid removal, it may have been a rare case in which Graves' disease (autoimmune caused hyperthyroidism) resolved without further treatment. It may also be that your case was actually that of Hashimoto's thyroiditis (autoimmune caused hypothyroidism) which can first present with a phase of hyperthyroidism - "Hashitoxicosis".

Your doctor could order tests for Anti-TPO and anti-TG antibodies and if one or both are positive, Hashimoto's would be a strong possibility. A tissue biopsy called an "FNA" (Fine Needle Aspiration) and a thyroid ultrasound would help confirm this as well, plus the latter one can help detect whether any thyroid nodules are present. The type called "hot nodules" can also be a cause of hyperthyroidism.

The Eltroxin drug you are now being treated with, is a thyroid hormone replacement drug. Many Thyroid Specialists and Endocrinologists suggest getting the TSH level (a blood hormone level most often used to monitor thyroid hormone replacement) suppressed down to between "1.0 and 2.0".

This is done to better optimized relief of hypothyroid symptoms (like fatigue). Some use "1.0" as their target treatment goal. These are things you might consider discussing with your doctor, to better understand your case."

Thyroid Eye Disease

When GD patients develop "Graves' Ophthalmopathy" (GO), this will also need to be treated. GO is a co-occurring inflammatory condition affecting the eyes (also called Thyroid Eye Disease). It can potentially develop in GD patients and can cause bulging of the eyes and possible deterioration of vision.

The most common treatments for GO include:

• *Eye drops to keep the eyes lubricated*

• *Corticosteroid therapy (steroid anti-inflammatory)*

• *Radiotherapy and/or Decompression Therapy to reduce orbital damage*

• *Eyelid surgery, to lengthen eyelids that may not cover the eyes well, due to them bulging.*

- - -

• *GD patients who smoke are sometimes also recommended by their doctors to quit smoking because of the inflammatory chemicals contained in cigarettes that can potentially affect the eyes.*

These are general overviews in regard to symptoms, diagnosis and treatments for Hashimoto's thyroiditis and Grave's Disease. Patients who are suspected of having either of these diseases must be evaluated or treated by a licensed physician. Thyroid Specializing MDs and Endocrinologists are the preferred types of physicians for treating diseases of thyroid autoimmunity.

CHAPTER FIVE

What are Goiters?

When a thyroid patient has a goiter, this simply
means they have swelling of the thyroid gland,
which is located at the front of the neck, in the
area just below the Adam's apple. The gland is
about the same size as the Adam's apple but has
two lobes on both sides, with the middle portion
(isthmus) being in the center, giving it a butterfly
shape. Goiters are recognized as different types
and as affecting part of the thyroid, such as one of
the two lobes or the isthmus or affecting the entire
gland as a whole (diffuse). They are also
considered different types depending upon the
causes of them.

Self-Examining for Goiters

While a person can sometimes detect a goiter
and/or thyroid nodules by self examination, a
definitive diagnoses must be given by a qualified
physician.

These abnormalities in size and/or texture of the
thyroid gland can occur with both hypothyroid
and hyperthyroid conditions.

They are however, more common in autoimmune thyroid diseases. If a person feels he may be experiencing thyroid-related symptoms or has detected an abnormal feeling in his thyroid, a preliminary self-examination can be done while an appointment with a qualified physician has been scheduled. A patient can then report any findings that indicate problems in the gland to his medical doctor. The emedicine/WebMD website states in their article titled "*Goiter Nontoxic: Follow-Up*", under the "Patient Education" sub-heading that "Thyroid self-examination, may be taught to patients, allowing them to monitor their own body for early changes in gland size."

Palpating the Thyroid Gland - A person can feel his own throat, using the fingertips (palpation), in the area of the thyroid gland, to detect swelling or lumps. The thyroid is located in the center of the throat, directly beneath the Adams apple, which in males is more prominent but can usually be located easily in females as well. Once finding the Adams apple, the isthmus (middle portion) of the thyroid is only about an inch or, slightly lower below it and will be slightly raised.

If the isthmus protrudes significantly, or feels very firm to the touch, this can indicate a goiter in that portion of the gland.

Shape of the Gland - There are also two lobes of the thyroid gland, one of each side of it, that extend about an inch toward the inside of the throat and that extend upward toward the Adams apple, about even with it. The gland is typically small and forms a butterfly shape. The lobes actually attach to the Adams apple and throat with connecting cartilage and tissue but when they are normal size, are usually not easily felt unless pressed-on firmly with the fingertips. If they are easily detectable without firmly pressing down on them or are visible without the need to palpate them, this can indicate a goiter or nodules in the lobe-areas as well.

The Swallow Test - While palpation is being done to detect swelling (enlargement) in the gland, any lumps or protrusions that might indicate a thyroid nodule (tumor-like growth) or several of them should also be checked for. These can also be spotted by tilting the head back, while looking in a mirror and taking sips of water.

This is done to watch for any signs of enlargement or lumps as the gland moves up and down in the throat. Some people with enlarged glands are found to have both goiter and nodules, which is referred to as a "nodular goiter" or a "multi-nodular goiter".

Difficulty Swallowing - If a person feels a lump on the inside of his throat when swallowing, this can indicate a thyroid nodule that is growing toward the inside and that cannot be felt from the outside of the throat. If there is a general feeling of difficulty swallowing or breathing due to the throat being constricted, this may also indicate a goiter in which the enlargement is swelling toward the inside of the throat. This type problem is not always indicative of thyroid problems but can be related to esophagus problems as well.

How Goiters are Medically Detected/Diagnosed

Patients, who have goiters or are suspected of having them, may be referred for a "thyroid ultrasound" (sound-wave imaging/sonogram) or a "thyroid uptake scan" (radiology/radioactive iodine) and possibly even an MRI (Magnetic Resonance Imaging).

These are diagnostic tests that give detailed images of the thyroid gland, to determine the size of goiters and whether they contain nodules (tumors) within them that are not detectable by palpation.

Types of Goiters

A major cause of goiters, are autoimmune thyroid diseases as previously described. If a person's thyroid gland has swelling plus a number of small nodules within it, they refer to this type as a "multi-nodular goiter". The nodules within a gland that has goiter can be the type that causes the thyroid gland to produce excess thyroid hormone, in which case, they will add the term "toxic" to the term, calling it a "toxic multi-nodular goiter".

People with Hashimoto's thyroiditis, commonly have multi-nodular goiters that are non-toxic. When a person is termed as having a "diffuse goiter", this means there is general swelling throughout the gland that is not caused by nodules.

This type of goiter can also cause toxicity or over-activity of the thyroid gland (hyperthyroidism), in which case it is referred to as a "toxic diffuse goiter". These types are found commonly in patients with Grave's Disease, as are toxic multi-nodular goiters.

If a goiter is caused by iodine deficiency, it is referred to as a "colloid nodular" or "endemic' goiter. This type is rare in the U.S. and other industrialized countries that use iodized table salt, which usually provides those that consume it, enough iodine to avoid iodine deficiency hypothyroidism and the resulting endemic goiters.

Temporary types of thyroiditis, such as those that occur with viral infections and in pregnant women can also cause goiter (transient asymmetrical enlargement) but these type will resolve within a few weeks, along with the thyroiditis. These type goiters can flare up short term with these types of thyroiditis and cause severe pain in the thyroid gland, which is referred to as "sub-acute thyroiditis", while others types do not cause a painful thyroid which is referred to as "silent thyroiditis".

CHAPTER SIX

What are Thyroid Nodules?

Thyroid nodules are small tumor-like growths on the thyroid gland as mentioned in the previous chapter. According to statistics, as much as 10 percent of the population has thyroid nodules but they occur far more often in people with thyroid diseases. People with thyroid autoimmunity have abnormal thyroid tissue and over time they can develop a large number of nodules or what is referred to as "multi-nodules".

How Thyroid Nodules are Detected/Diagnosed

Thyroid nodules can be detected by feel or "palpation" just as goiters can but some may be in an area of the gland that are only detectable by diagnostic imaging tests such as "thyroid ultrasound" (sound wave imaging), "Radio Active Iodine Uptake Scans" (radiological imaging) and "MRI" (Magnetic Resonance Imaging).

Thyroid nodules that are solitary or found to be a single one, rather than found among a group of them have a slightly higher risk.

These type may contain cancer cells (malignancy) than do multi-nodules and larger nodules are also considered more suspicious. When a solitary nodule is located, the treating Doctor may wish to have a tissue biopsy performed to see if it contains malignant cells.

The procedure that is usually performed to obtain a thyroid nodule tissue sample is called a "Fine Needle Aspiration" (FNA) and is a simple out-patient procedure. The tissue sample is then lab-analyzed to detect any abnormal cells indicating the presence of either "papillary" or "follicular" cancer, which are the two major types that can potentially invade the thyroid gland.

Types of Thyroid Nodules

When thyroid nodules are being investigated, they may be placed into several categories. Two of the more basic categories of thyroid nodules, are those that are solitary (single ones) and multi-nodules (a group of several). Other types include hot nodules that actively absorb iodine from the thyroid gland, releasing thyroid hormone, causing a hormone imbalance in the patient (hyperthyroidism).

Smaller hot nodules may not cause hyperthyroidism while larger ones usually do and many times are also biopsied due to their larger size. If the nodule is not resulting in increased thyroid hormone release, it is referred to as a "cold nodule" and both hot and cold nodules have a distinct appearance on diagnostic imaging tests.

Some thyroid nodules are more solid than others which are referred to as a "solid nodules" and these are also considered more suspicious of possibly containing cancer cells (as large ones are) and may also be biopsied as a precaution, depending upon their size. Many non-solid nodules are considered to be "cystic nodules" because they will contain fluid in the center of them and these type, are almost never considered a risk for containing cancer cells.

Treatment for Goiters and Thyroid Nodules

The most common treatment for both goiters and benign thyroid nodules is thyroid hormone replacement therapy. Treating doctors will prescribe a dose of thyroid hormone that can help to shrink goiters and nodules over time and can also prevent further growth of them.

If a goiter or thyroid nodule is large enough to
obstruct a patient's breathing or swallowing, a
treating doctor might refer the patient for surgery,
to remove a nodule or part of the thyroid gland
and possibly all of it.

In cases of malignancy found in the thyroid gland,
total thyroid removal is always the treatment.
Afterward the patient must have thyroid hormone
replacement therapy for the rest of their lives.
More in regard to malignant thyroid conditions
will be discussed in the next chapter addressing
thyroid cancer.

CHAPTER SEVEN

Thyroid Cancer

Of all the thyroid disorders and diseases that exist, thyroid cancer is the least common of them all but at the same time is increasing faster than any other form of cancer.

Thyroid cancer should be taken very seriously as should any form of cancer because any type that is not diagnosed and treated in time has the potential to spread to other parts of the body via the lymph nodes found near the thyroid gland.

According to medical research on thyroid cancer, chances of developing it are increased in people with a family history of thyroid cancer.

At the same time, thyroid cancer has a very high treatment success rate and that success rate is increased when early diagnosis and treatment is administered.

According to medical sources, only about 5% of thyroid nodules are found to contain cancer

How Thyroid Cancer Manifests

Thyroid cancers always present as thyroid nodules (tumors) in the thyroid gland but some tumors are more easily recognizable than others.

To repeat: Some thyroid nodules may require an FNA (tissue biopsy) when they are of a certain size that makes them suspicious of possibly containing malignancy or cancer cells. The same is true if nodules are found to be solid, meaning they are not typical nodules that are softer in texture (warm nodules) or cystic but are very firm, which are also sometimes referred to as "cold nodules". Single nodules are also considered more suspicious than are multi-nodules, meaning several of them, rather than a single one and might also have FNA biopsies ordered to evaluate them. While an FNA can detect certain types of cancers that affect the thyroid gland, other types, such as carcinomas need surgical biopsies performed to detect them. More about the FNA test will be discussed in the next subheading in regard to diagnosing thyroid cancer.

Some types of thyroid cancer tumors, take on the appearance of thyroid gland tissue which means they are less malignant and more treatable. The type, that resemble thyroid tissue are referred to as "differentiated". Other types have a distinctly different appearance from normal thyroid tissue and these types are referred to as "undifferentiated" and have a higher malignancy rate and are sometimes more difficult to treat.

Many thyroid tumors (nodules) are found incidentally, when a person happens to detect one by feel or they may feel a lump on the inside of their throat when swallowing. When the patient sees their doctor, he may palpate (feel) the nodule to see if it feels firm or of significant size. If he finds that the nodule needs further investigation, he may refer the patient for testing.

Sometimes, a thyroid nodule will grow toward the inside of the throat, and the person will feel it as a lump when swallowing. If the nodule is malignant, and it is an aggressive type of cancer, the nodule can grow large enough to obstruct breathing and swallowing over time.

How Thyroid Cancer is Diagnosed

There are a number of procedures used to diagnose thyroid cancer, including blood tests to detect highly elevated levels of thyroglobulin, cancer cells (new advancements) and for the presence of "Calcitonin" (found with medullary cancer). Imaging tests may also be ordered, including a Thyroid Ultrasound, CT Scans, MRIs and 24 hour Thyroid Uptake Scans.

The single most diagnostic test to detect the presence of thyroid cancer, are biopsies of the affected thyroid tissue. This includes using a fine needle to extract tissue samples and surgical biopsies when larger tissue samples are needed.

An FNA is performed using a needle that is inserted into the patient's thyroid gland and tissue from the gland or nodules being biopsied, is extracted and sent for laboratory analysis. While it is a fairly non-evasive procedure, patients should expect some soreness for a few days following the procedure. The fine needle that is used does not leave scarring and a local anesthesia is used to numb the area on the neck, before the needle is inserted.

Thyroid Cancer Treatment

When a patient is confirmed as having thyroid cancer, via the tests that diagnose it, the treating doctor will refer the patient to a surgeon, who will determine how the cancer will need to be removed. If the cancer affects only one of the two lobes of the thyroid, the surgeon may wish to perform what is called a "lobectomy", (partial thyroidectomy) meaning there will be removal of only one side of the gland.

If the surgeon feels removal of only one lobe, still places the patient at risk for the cancer returning, he may instead decide to remove the entire gland, which is referred to as a "total thyroidectomy". The type surgery is also determined by considering the type of thyroid cancer that is involved. Some types of cancer are more aggressive than others and with these the surgeon will always recommend total thyroid removal. Surgeons also must determine at what stage the cancer is in, meaning how far it has progressed.

In order to decrease the risk of the cancer returning, the surgeon may also want to remove the lymph nodes in the neck, that are located near the thyroid gland.

The lymph nodes may also be sent off for laboratory analysis to determine if they already contained cancer, which might then lead the surgeon to recommend further treatment(s).

Post Operative Thyroid Cancer Treatments

Additional treatment after any type of thyroidectomy might also include Radio Active Iodine Therapy (RAI) or Chemotherapy, to destroy any remaining thyroid tissue that is capable of absorbing iodine in the body or any remaining cancer cells. Any remaining thyroid tissue that is capable of taking up iodine, which is what the thyroid mainly consists of, also has the ability to re-develop cancer cells and is the reason RAI is sometimes used following a Total Thyroidectomy. Chemotherapy is directed at any remaining cancer cells that might remain in the body after a Total Thyroidectomy.

Regardless of the type of thyroid surgery that is performed, thyroid hormone replacement therapy is always used following thyroid cancer surgeries. The goal of the hormone therapy is to suppress the patient's TSH level, which decreases when thyroid hormone is increased via a hormone dose.

This also helps prevent recurrence of cancer but also replaces any hormone the thyroid gland is not capable of producing following surgery (hypothyroidism).

If a patient is given RAI after surgery, they may not be replaced with thyroid hormone for a month or two following the treatment. Most patients will need thyroid hormone replacement therapy following any type of thyroidectomy, as lifelong treatment.

The treating Doctor will prescribe a starting dose of thyroid hormone for the patient and will order follow-up blood re-testing to adjust the dose to the correct level over time, which is called "titrating" the dose. Each new dose level takes about eight weeks to fully adjust in the body.

Following are helpful suggestions for patients who are placed on thyroid hormone therapy following thyroid cancer treatment:

• *Take your thyroid hormone medication on an empty stomach, with plenty of water.*

• *Take your thyroid hormone medication at the same time each day.*

- - -

• *If you take vitamins or supplements containing iron or calcium, be sure to take them six hours apart from your thyroid medication dose.*

• *When you have blood retests of your thyroid hormone levels, take your medication at the same time, to correlate with each blood draw.*

• *Never adjust your own thyroid medication dose.*

Thyroid cancers have a very high treatment success rate as previously mentioned but that success rate is even higher when thyroid cancers are diagnosed and treated as early as possible.

It is very important to see your doctor if you discover any nodules (tumor-like growths) on your thyroid gland or if you have difficulty swallowing or feel, that you might have a growth on the inside of your throat.

It is also important to seek medical evaluation as soon as possible, if you experience the symptoms of either an overactive or under active thyroid gland.

(END)